DYSTONIA

IDEAS FOR PREVENTING DYSTONIA

DR. MONTANA CANNON

Table of Contents

CHAPTER ONE

INTRODUCTION

Dystonia is a movement ailment that reasons the muscular tissues to contract involuntarily. This may cause repetitive or twisting movements.

The circumstance may have an impact on one part of your body (focal dystonia), or more adjacent elements (segmental dystonia), or all factors of your frame (preferred dystonia). The muscle spasms can range from mild to intense. They'll be painful, and they're capable of interfere together with your performance of every day responsibilities.

There is no therapy for dystonia, however medications and treatment can enhance symptoms. Surgical procedure is from time to time used to disable or regulate nerves or sure brain areas in people with immoderate dystonia.

Dystonia is a situation where a person has uncontrollable muscle actions in a few a part of their frame. This happens because of faulty signs coming from their thoughts. Dystonia can range from a quick-time period or brief project to a lifelong trouble. Most instances are treatable, especially instances with a treatable or curable underlying cause.

Dystonia is a worried system disorder that motives uncontrollable muscle contractions, which means a person's muscle mass worrying up with out seeking to make the muscle organizations do so. Even though it affects muscles, it's clearly an problem in conjunction with your brain or each different part of your anxious system.

The decision "dystonia" is a mixture of the Latin prefix "dys-," and the Greek word "-tonos," which refers to muscle anxiety. The mixture of the two terms describes a trouble wherein your muscle groups worrying up in a manner that's defective or incorrect.

Dystonia is a movement disease in which a person's muscle mass contract uncontrollably. The contraction causes the affected frame detail to curve involuntarily, ensuing in repetitive actions or odd postures. Dystonia may have an effect on one muscle, a muscle organization, or the complete body. Dystonia influences approximately 1% of the populace, and girls are more liable to it than guys.

Dystonia is a illness that impacts the way the frame moves. It causes the muscle tissues to settlement, which makes them flow involuntarily or get stuck in an strange characteristic. Dystonia can affect the entire frame or a positive detail, and the movements can sometimes cause ache.

What is the difference amongst dystonia and dyskinesia?

Dyskinesia and dystonia are intently related but aren't the same.

Dyskinesia: This phrase comes from Greek.

"Kinesia" comes from the word "kinesis," which means that that "movement." The combined phrase refers to movements which may be defective or appear in a manner they should not. Dyskinesias are involuntary muscle actions, which means you do no longer manage that they're occurring.

Dystonia. That is a selected form of dyskinesia. With dystonia, muscle corporations worrying up for longer durations. Depending on what a part of your frame they show up in, they could frequently reason you to transport or pose in tremendous strategies.

Who does dystonia have an impact on?

Counting on why it occurs, all and sundry

can boom dystonia. Some reasons are age-particular, affecting humans at starting or in adolescence, at the identical time as others are more likely to expand late in existence.

How does dystonia have an effect on my frame?

Dystonia is a mind situation that affects how your mind controls muscles for the duration of your frame. This could have an effect on muscle mass or businesses of muscle groups in specific techniques. Exactly how and why this occurs remains a thriller, even though. The effects of dystonia can also get worse whilst you experience worn-out or compelled, or if you drink caffeine or alcohol.

Some varieties of dystonia happen because of genetic mutations or conditions that disrupt the manner additives of your thoughts work. This will cause the affected cells to paintings incorrectly, predominant to faulty signals engaging in your muscle groups and causing dystonia's outcomes.

Dystonia also can show up because of injuries or conditions that disrupt your brain feature, and some of the ones situations are visible on imaging scans or detectable with positive tests. But it can additionally show up for exclusive motives.

Signs

Dystonia impacts exquisite people in unique approaches. Muscle spasms would probably:

Begin in a unmarried vicinity, inclusive of your leg, neck or arm. Focal dystonia that starts after age 21 generally starts offevolved inside the neck, arm or face. It has a tendency to live focal or grow to be segmental.

Rise up in some unspecified time in the future of a particular movement, together with writing by the use of hand.

Get worse with stress, fatigue or anxiety.

Come to be extra predominant through the years.

Regions of the body that can be affected embody:

Neck (cervical dystonia). Contractions reason your head to curve and flip to one factor, or pull ahead or backward, from time to time inflicting ache.

Eyelids. Rapid blinking or spasms cause your eyes to close (blepharospasms) and make it difficult as a way to see. Spasms generally aren't painful however might likely boom at the same time as you are in shiny mild, studying, looking television, under pressure or interacting with humans. Your eyes could probably enjoy dry, gritty or sensitive to slight.

Jaw or tongue (oromandibular dystonia). You could enjoy slurred speech, drooling, and hassle chewing or swallowing. Oromandibular dystonia can be painful and regularly occurs in mixture with cervical dystonia or blepharospasm.

Voice container and vocal cords (laryngeal dystonia). You would possibly have a very good or whispering voice.

Hand and forearm. Some kinds of dystonia arise simplest while you do a repetitive pastime, which includes writing (writer's dystonia) or gambling a specific musical tool (musician's dystonia). Signs typically do not take place at the same time as your arm is at rest.

Whilst to peer a medical doctor

Early signs and symptoms of dystonia regularly are mild, occasional and related to a selected interest. See your health care provider in case you're having involuntary muscle contractions.

CHAPTER TWO

The exact motive of dystonia isn't always seemed. But it might incorporate adjustments in communication between nerve cells in severa areas of the mind. A few varieties of dystonia are exceeded down in households.

Dystonia can also be a symptom of any other disorder or scenario, together with:

Parkinson's ailment

Huntington's sickness

Wilson's ailment

Stressful brain damage

Shipping damage

Stroke

Mind tumor or certain troubles that growth in a few people with most cancers (paraneoplastic syndromes)

Oxygen deprivation or carbon monoxide poisoning

Infections, alongside tuberculosis or encephalitis

Reactions to certain medicinal drugs or heavy steel poisoning

Headaches

Relying on the kind of dystonia, headaches

can embody:

Physical disabilities that affect your common performance of each day activities or unique responsibilities

Hassle with imaginative and prescient that influences your eyelids

Trouble with jaw movement, swallowing or speech

Ache and fatigue, because of steady contraction of your muscle companies

Melancholy, tension and social withdrawal

How is dystonia recognized?

A healthcare issuer, frequently a neurologist, can diagnose dystonia based in your signs, a neurological examination and diverse medical assessments. Diagnosing dystonia is frequently intricate because its signs can seem with such a whole lot of one of a kind conditions. Which means it's important to rule out those other conditions, some of which may be life-threatening scientific emergencies.

What tests could be executed to diagnose dystonia?

A significant type of lab, diagnostic and imaging tests are feasible with dystonia. The most possibly checks rely on your symptoms and what conditions healthcare providers suspect. Feasible assessments consist of, but aren't restrained to, the following:

Blood checks (those can discover many problems, beginning from immune tool problems to pollutants and poisons, especially metals like copper or manganese).

Automatic tomography (CT) experiment.

Electroencephalogram (EEG).

Electromyogram (nerve conduction take a look at).

Genetic trying out.

Magnetic resonance imaging (MRI).

Positron emission tomography (puppy) test.

Spinal faucet (lumbar puncture).

Different exams are feasible, so your healthcare issuer is the fine individual to ask about the assessments they suggest in your specific case. The information they provide might be the maximum accurate in your instances.

How is dystonia dealt with, and is there a remedy?

There's no way to treatment dystonia, however it is probably treatable. Many possible remedies rely upon the underlying purpose or situation, or the signs and signs you've got were given. Your healthcare provider is the first rate man or woman to tell you the treatment options they advocate on your precise scenario.

Is there some thing i can't devour or drink with dystonia?

Your healthcare issuer might also additionally advocate which you keep away from caffeine and alcohol. For some people, consuming beverages that incorporate both could make dystonia signs and symptoms and symptoms worse.

What medicines or treatments are used?

The feasible drug treatments or remedies for dystonia depend upon why it's happening and the specific signs and symptoms you've got were given. In wellknown, the following treatment types are possible:

Deep mind stimulation. This remedy involves surgical remedy to implant electrodes into your brain. Those electrodes supply a mild electrical present day to a part of your mind, that could assist the symptoms of dystonia. That is the maximum not unusual and maximum useful surgical treatment for dystonia.

Medicinal capsules. Counting on why dystonia takes place, it's often feasible to deal with it with medicinal drug. The medicine (or combination of them) is based upon at the signs and symptoms and the underlying purpose — if there is one — of the dystonia.

Botulinum toxin injections. Botulinum toxin — usually regarded beneath the trademarked name Botox® — can block all nerve indicators for weeks or even months when injected in the proper location. That maintains the alerts that purpose dystonia from getting on your muscle mass, making botulinum toxin a treatment choice for focal or a few segmental dystonia signs.

Bodily, occupational and speech therapy. Those varieties of remedy can frequently help a person adapt or get over dystonia, mainly while dystonia takes place because of a transient health situation or situation.

Headaches/component outcomes of remedy

The headaches and aspect outcomes feasible with dystonia rely upon numerous elements, beginning with the remedies themselves. Your healthcare company is the splendid person to offer an explanation for what's possible or in all likelihood for you due to the fact they are able to give you records that considers your occasions.

How do I take care of myself or manage signs and symptoms and symptoms?

Dystonia is a neurological trouble, which means that it isn't a few issue you can self-diagnose and self-treat. It's additionally important to talk for your healthcare provider earlier than later due to the fact dystonia can show up with severe or existence-threatening situations.

How soon after remedy will I experience higher, and the manner prolonged does it take to get better?

The timeline at the manner to experience higher and get higher depends on why your dystonia happened, how severe it is, the remedies you acquired, some other health situations you could have and extra. Your healthcare issuer is the great individual to tell you approximately the probably timeline for you to experience better and recover.

How am i able to lessen my risk or save you dystonia altogether?

Dystonia happens unpredictably, so that you can't save you it. You can also't reduce the chance of developing primary dystonia. That's due to the fact you both inherit it or increase it for unknown reasons.

But, some reasons of secondary dystonia are preventable, or you can reduce your hazard of growing them. The matters you could do include:

Devour a balanced diet and hold a healthful weight. Many conditions related to your circulatory and heart fitness, mainly stroke, can damage areas of your thoughts, inflicting dystonia. Stopping, delaying or reducing the severity of those situations may have a big effect on whether or not or not or not you expand dystonia.

Don't ignore infections. Eye and ear infections need rapid treatment. Even as the ones infections spread to your mind, they grow to be a intense chance. Infections can cause mind contamination (encephalitis) that would result in dystonia.

Put on protection device. Annoying mind accidents can damage your brain and purpose dystonia. That makes protection device vital in decreasing your danger of developing this situation.

Manipulate your health situations. Continual conditions cause or contribute to other situations that reason dystonia. That includes situations like kind 2 diabetes, high blood stress, epilepsy and others.

How do I contend with myself?

If you have dystonia, there may be some matters you may do to attend to your self, which includes:

Keep away from caffeine and alcohol in case your healthcare issuer recommends this. Those can make dystonia signs and symptoms worse.

Manage your pressure. Anxiety and pressure can purpose dystonia to get worse. You may reduce this threat by means of handling your stress and anxiety with strategies like meditation, relaxation schooling, workout and extra.

Avoid sports that make symptoms worse. Some varieties of dystonia are much more likely to occur below certain events. Avoiding those instances, at the same time as possible, can lessen the opportunities of dystonia symptoms and signs and symptoms flaring up.

Discover ways to manage your circumstance. One in every of a kind forms of dystonia are often potential with "sensory recommendations." A key time period for that is "geste antagoniste," it truly is French for "hostile gesture." An adversarial gesture can reason dystonia signs to get better quickly, even though specialists don't recognise precisely why this takes place. An instance of an hostile gesture is touching your chin or the thing of your face to help relieve the signs and symptoms of cervical dystonia (which influences muscle groups to your head and neck). Your healthcare business enterprise can help find in case you reply to those gestures and train you the way to use them.

Take your remedy. In case you take medicinal drug for dystonia, take your remedy as prescribed. All of sudden preventing your remedy can get worse dystonia symptoms and signs and symptoms or reason one of a kind component outcomes.

If you have dystonia, you have to see your healthcare corporation for examine-up visits as encouraged. You need to additionally see them if your symptoms and symptoms exchange or worsen, in particular if the modifications disrupt your life and normal. Also see them if medicinal tablets or exclusive remedies lose effectiveness or purpose side outcomes which can be hard to cope with or disruptive.

CONCLUSION

Dystonia is a thoughts situation that reasons defective alerts in your muscular tissues, which makes those muscle mass move uncontrollably. This situation can show up for many reasons, beginning from lifelong inherited situations to brief-time period illnesses. The severity of the symptoms and symptoms and the manner remarkable the outcomes are on your frame could make this circumstance a minor inconvenience, or they can be appreciably disruptive and keep you from doing sure matters.

While it isn't curable, dystonia is regularly treatable, mainly with high quality motives. In some instances, dystonia may fit away completely while it occurs with quick-term or curable conditions.

THE END